Red Maca

Combat Infertility, Boost Your Immune System and Reclaim Your Energy, Sex Drive and Women Dillodo. (The Raw Red Maca Root Powder, Gelatinized and Peruvian)

Dionisia Onio

Table of Contents

INTRODUCTION

Have you wondered how to add natural ingredients into your daily life to give you maximum benefits? Do you struggle with hormonal imbalances, fatigue, and problems sleeping? Do you look for pharmaceutical relief but continue to stress your life away? Take a little bit of your time to learn the benefits Red Maca has to offer you.

If you have been curious about adding Red Maca to your diet, it is time to stop wondering. Take advantage of this potent herb and challenge yourself to fully understand the amazing benefits of a natural substance. Challenge yourself to make Red Maca a part of your daily life and see the results months or even weeks from now. This book covers scientific research and anonymous testimonials that people have stated after making use of Red Maca.

Infertility is characterized as powerlessness of a couple to conceive after 12 months of unprotected sexual intercourse. It affects over five million couples alone in the U. S. and furthermore commonly to all the more on the planet. Due to unawareness of medicines, just 10% looks for assistance from expert authority.

Maca root like radish roots, comes from Peru, and flourishes at altitudes over 4,000 meters. A large number of scientists around the globe, have paid more consideration to the investigation of the properties and impacts of this plant. Maca root has been used by the indigenous people of Peru as a pharmaceutical and nourishment source through the year 2000. They likewise utilize it to support and turns barrenness, extraordinarily improves power, sexual genuinely and vitality.

You deserve a quality life. Invest in a quality root vegetable that has been around since ancient times. See what the rants and raves are about Red Maca and why it is still around today. **What You Will Discover:**

- What Red Maca is?

- Essential information about the maca root

- Benefits of the root

- Using the maca root to enhance fertility

- Research conducted on the maca root

- Where you can purchase the amazing herb

- Side effects of the maca root and many more...

CHAPTER 1

What Is Red Maca?

Red Maca (lepidium meyenii or lepidium peruvianum) is the second rarest of all varieties of maca, making up about 25% of the yearly harvest. It is sometimes referred to as pink or purple Maca, however is most generally known as "Red Maca." It grows in the regions and under similar conations as other more common types of Maca and yet has some unique properties that are quick making it the Maca of preference. During the last few years it has gain quite a bit of popularity and quite without a doubt, once we tried it 2 years ago, it has become our favorite variety not only because of the increased efficiency, but also because of the taste.

How is Red Maca Different?

If you were to visit a Maca farm, before the roots are made right into a powder, you'd quickly and without difficulty be able to tell the difference between Red Maca, Yellow/Cream Maca and Black Maca. As you can see from the images right here, every of the roots are of a special shade – and on this way they're named.

Even though all organically grown high quality Maca powders shares a nearly equal dietary profile, Red Maca has been shown, under phytonutrient analysis, to be higher in certain compounds that supports the body in antioxidant and antitumoral activity. It has been show amongst all Maca colors to contain somewhat higher levels of other pythonutrients which includes alkaloids, tannins, saponis and steroids.

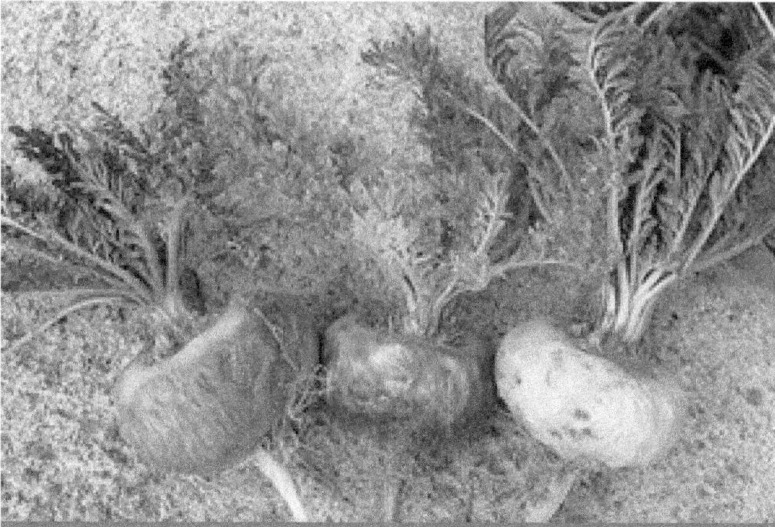

RED, BLACK AND YELLOW MACA ROOTS

Another substantial difference between Red Maca and Cream or Black Maca is the taste. The majority find the taste to be gentle and mild. We've found that to be true as well and might describe the taste as similar to a subtle caramel. One of my clients lately wrote me to allow me to know that her kids love Red Maca on their oatmeal in preference to sugar as it tastes so sweet!

What Studies Have Been Carried Out On Red Maca?

Interest in Maca amongst medical professionals is growing as are research studies. In terms of studies on Red Maca powder particularly, there are three main tremendous ones.

1. The most vital study done on Red Maca was published in the journal reproductive Biology and endocrinology 2005; 3:5. In it 8 medical researchers report that over the course of 42 days: "Red Maca however neither Yellow/Cream nor Black Maca reduced significantly ventral prostate size in rats." the studies also goes on to document that under pyhtochemical analysis for 7 RED-Web functional nutrient groups, "Highest peak were observed for Red Maca, intermediate values for Yellow/Cream Maca and low values for Black Maca."

2. In 2010 researchers from the Universidad Peruana, Lima published a study on the effects of Maca on bone structure in rats that had had their ovaries removed. The conclusion was that both "Red and Black Maca have protective effects on bone architecture in OVX rats without showing estrogenic effects on uterine weight."

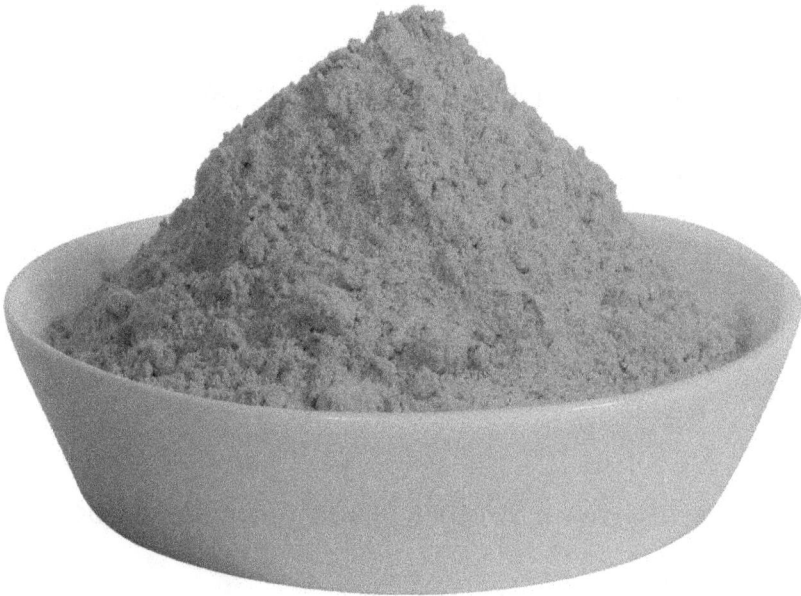

3. Finally another study from the same University in 2009 found that Black Maca to increase sperm production more than Yellow or Red Maca. The study

concluded that while Red Maca, like other Maca's, had a favorable effect on energy, mood and sexual desire, it did little to increase the volume of sperm produced in comparison to Black or Yellow Maca.

How Can Red Maca Support Vibrant Health?

Red Maca, just like the Yellow/Cream and Black Maca can do all the following:

- Boost overall energy and vitality

- Balance hormones for both women and men – this can support with menopause, pimples, fertility, thyroid and other health problems associated with the endocrine system.

- Support a healthy libido and sex drive.

Similarly Red Maca mainly appears to be the best colors for :

- Prostate protection – most important for men and in particular men over 40

- Bone density – most important for women and children

Complete Dietary Breakdown Of Red Maca

Sample length 100g:

Carbohydrates 62.6g, fats 0.82g, fiber 5.3g, protein 17.9g

Protein components (%): Albumins & Globulins 74, Glutelins 15.3, Prolamins 10.6, True protein 42.1

Vitamin & minerals (mg %): Ascorbic acid 3.52, Boron 12, Calcium 490, Iron 80, Magnesium 70, Niacin 43, Phosphorous 320, Potassium 113, Riboflavin 0.61, Sodium 20, Thiamine 0.42, Zinc 12.

Amino Acids: Alanine 63.1, Arginine 99.4, Asparatic Acid 91.7, Red Maca PowderGlutamatic Acid 156, Glycine 68.3, HO-Proline 26, Hystidine 21.9, Isoleucine

47.4, Leucine 91, Lysine 54.5 Methionine 28, Phenylalanine 55.3 Proline 0.5, Sarcosine 0.7, Serine 50.4, Threonine 33.1, Tyrosine 30.6, Valine 79.3

Final Thought On Red Maca - Raw Vs. Gelatinized

I love all kinds of Maca and have enjoyed the benefits of them for years. I like to use variety of Maca colors for myself and normally have Cream, Red and Black Maca on hand. That said, my favorite tasting Maca is Red Maca. I highly recommend it as it offers nearly all the advantages of the other forms of Maca with the exception of increasing sperm count.

Major marketers now sell Red Maca in both raw and gelatinized bureaucracy. For most people i recommend the raw product as all of it's nutrients are 100% intact. However, when you have a sensitive stomach or an issues with digesting starch you're better off getting the gelatinized product.

CHAPTER 2

What Is Yellow Maca?

Maca root powder is a loved a part of life in the high Andes. Yellow Maca is the most common of all colors, making up about 60% of the annual harvest. Ours is made from roots traditionally grown and harvested on an organic farming co-op in a remote pristine part of the Peruvian Andes. It is never heated above 106 degrees F in an effort to preserve nutrients at maximum levels. Yellow Maca has been the most researched of all three maca colors.

- Yellow Maca is nutrient dense with 60% carbohydrates, 12 crucial minerals, 10 vitamins, over 40 fatty and amino acids and 4 unique glucosinolates – a true superfood.

- Used for over 2000 years as a nutritionally dense food to promote endurance, vitality, fertility and libido in populations living at very high elevations.

- Grown in the Andes at elevations above 14000 feet and in extreme cold, wind and sunlight, Maca is the world's highest growing crop

- As Yellow Maca is the most common Maca it's also the least expensive.

Yellow Maca Root Powder Is:

- Certified Organic

- GMO Free

- Fair Trade

- Grown traditionally with respect for the land - near Junin, Peru

- Sun dried, carefully processed and packaged

without delay

- 100% Raw and Vegan

- Contain Only Yellow Maca Root Powder

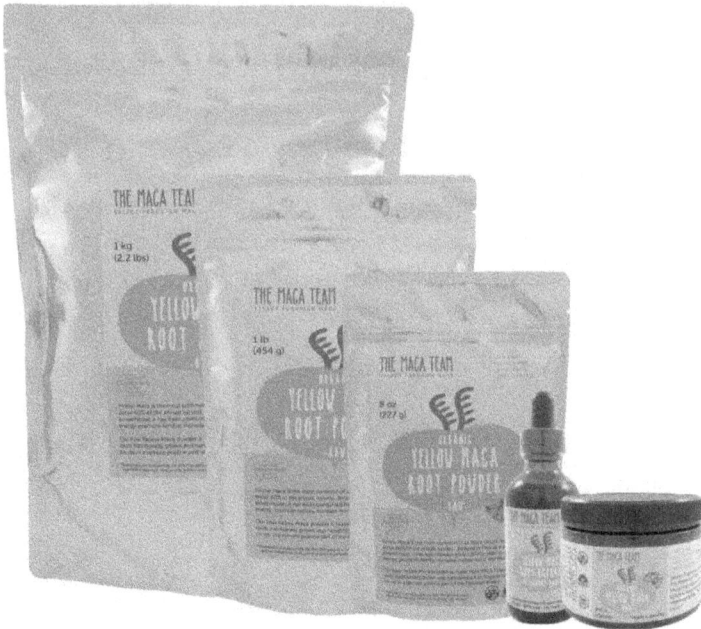

Yellow Maca Powder Is A Great Way To Begin With Maca.

To this point loads of researches, all available publicly in the pubmed database, has found it to be useful for energy building, fertile, hormone stability or balance, mental awareness and more. Yellow Maca is certainly a nutritional powerhouse, containing nearly all essential amino acids and free fatty acids, substantial levels of vitamins A, B1, B2, B3, and C, minerals iron, magnesium, zinc and calcium, a high concentration of bio-available protein and nutrients unique to Maca called *Macaenes* and *Macamides*. Maca is also an "*Adaptogen,*" or rare form of plant that is thought to elevate the overall life force energy of those who eat it.

Cream Maca Root Powder In 3 Sizes: (Servings Based Totally On 3 Tsp Or 9 g Every Day)

- 8 ounces (25 servings)
- 16 oz (50 servings)
- 1 kg - 35 ounces (111 servings) - exceptional price!

In vegan capsules

- 750 mg every, 2 hundred ct (28 servings)

And in glycerine based liquid extracts

2 fl oz (59ml)

CHAPTER 3

7 Things to Understand About Correct Maca Dosage

1. Maca is a food – initially, it's important to take into account that natural maca powder, whether gelatinized or raw is a meals. It comes from a turnip like root high in the Andes mountains and has been eaten for thousands of years by people and animals indigenous to the vicinity. Maca is in contrast to other foods, though, in that it's a true nutritional powerhouse and an adaptogen.

2. You can't overdose, but... – from my own experience it's pretty much impossible to take too much of Maca. (Since it's a food and not a drug, herb or supplement). That said, some people report increased coronary heart rate and nervous energy when they take too much. That's

why you need to start with a conservative amount and work your way up slowly.

3. You have to consider your body weight - whilst you're starting with Maca, you need to consider how much you weigh as an important factor in figuring out your dosage. The dosage levels i suggest beneath are for those who weigh 160 pounds (75 KG). Bigger people can generally take more. Smaller people need to start with a smaller quantity.

4. You should also consider your general health and age – after factoring in your weight, also reflect on your overall level of health and your age. A 30 year old athlete can start taking a higher Maca dosage than a 75 year old retiree. The younger and healthier you are the more you can begin with.

5. Maca affects different people differently – even factoring in age, health and body weight, it's important to

remember the fact that Maca has different effects on different people. No two bodies are exactly alike and for the reason that Maca is an adaptogen it will act in your body to support what your body needs to balance – particularly in terms of your hormonal system.

6. You may regulate quantities as needed – one thing that we do often hear is to adjust the amount of Maca we take depending on how much energy we need, or how long way we've come along in our health goals. Sometimes we'll even forestall taking Maca for some days, whilst we feel like a break – more of that during a minute.

7. Therapeutic Maca dosage is different than general health dosage – one very last consideration is that recommended dosages of Maca for therapeutic purpose are usually higher than for general health. For example if you are taking Maca in particular to help with fertility, you may need to boost your intake over time.

Maca Dosage Recommendations - Powder - Capsules - Extracts

These dosage levels are primarily based on a forty year old with generally good health and weighing 160 lbs. If you weigh more or less adjust the dosage accordingly. *Note:* 1 measuring teaspoon of Maca powder weighs 3 grams.

Raw Maca – all colors together with Red Maca, Black Maca and Yellow Maca

Daily Recommendations – 3-9 grams (1-3 teaspoons) or 2-8 capsules

Raw Premium Maca

Daily Recommendations – 3-6 grams (1-2 teaspoons) or 2-8 capsules

Gelatinized Maca – all colors such as Red, Black and Yellow Maca (note: despite the fact that Gelatinized Maca is more concentrated, I will advise the equal amount to make up for the fact that some nutrients were destroyed by heating it).

Daily Recommendations – 3-9 grams (1-3 teaspoons) or 2-8 capsules

Gelatinized Premium Maca

Daily Recommendations – 3-6 grams (1-2 teaspoons) or 2-8 tablets

Maca Extracts

Daily Recommendations – 2-4 droppersful (1/4-1/2 teaspoon)

CHAPTER 4

Maca For Women's Fertility

Women have been using Maca powder to increase their chances of conceiving a child for over 2000 years. Clinical studies have proven that maca balances hormones which leads to regular ovulation. Additionally, Maca is a nutritional powerhouse that supports the optimal health needed to boost fertility. Red Maca has been shown to be the best maca for women seeking to boost their fertility.

Maca For Pregnancy

Maca is taken into consideration and generally safe to take during pregnancy stage. In reality, because of its high nutrient and mineral content, it could support healthy development. A 2-teaspoon serving of maca has 3 times more calcium than a glass of milk. Additionally, Black and Red Maca have been seen to increase bone density and strength. That said, if you have any worries about taking maca while you are pregnant, please seek advice from a competent medical expert.

Maca For Healthy Skin

Due to Maca's ability to help balance hormones, it frequently has a positive effect on pores and skin tone. This may include reducing hormone related pimples as well as improving skin elasticity. All maca powders which include cream colored maca works properly for this benefit.

Maca For Increased Libido

One of the biggest effects said by women taking proper dosages of Maca powder daily is a marked increase in sexual desire. Red Maca is the type of Maca that is highest in phytontutrients and, not surprisingly, is the maca of choice to enhance female libido.

Maca For Hot Flashes And Other Menopause Symptoms

Maca works very well to reduce all uncomfortable signs and symptoms of menopause and perimenopause inclusive of insomnia, mood swings and specifically hot flashes. This effect comes from maca's high-quality capacity to support healthy hormone balance. Maca does not contain hormones, but merely stimulates the body to balance the endocrine system. Red Maca is the best for women passing through this life transition.

Maca For Hair Growth

Because of Maca's brilliant hormone balancing properties in combination with it's dense dietary content, the food is capable of stimulating hair growth in women who have thinning hair.

Maca For Reducing/Preventing Osteoperosis

Research have shown that Red and Black Maca were found to be the best at enhancing and protecting bone structure specifically in mice who had their ovaries removed. Other research have proven that maca increases bone strength and density.

Maca For Thyroid Health

Because of maca's hormone balancing properties, it has been suggested to have a positive effect on the health of the thyroid. Maca does contain iodine which affects the thyroid. If you have an iodine allergy you should avoid Maca.

Maca For Enhanced Curves

One of the more thrilling effects of Maca is that it can support the enhancement of female body shape. Maca works to balance estrogen levels, which can increase the size and shape of breasts. Additionally, considering the fact that Maca is extraordinarily anabolic (muscle building) it can increase the size of the buttocks, that which is of the body's largest muscle. If you want to get the most benefit for the latter, i recommend using Black Maca and also getting plenty of exercising aimed at increasing the glutes.

Maca For Women And Athletic Performance

Maca is exquisite for athletes. It builds muscle, it increases stamina, it boosts energy and it enhances recuperation time. Black Maca is my Maca of preference for athletes.

Maca For Reducing Depression

One of the lesser recognized benefits of Maca for women is for lowering depression. Maca works as a mood up-lifter because of its high nutrient content combined with its energizing properties. I've had numerous reports of positive emotional health resulting from continued use of Red Maca.

CHAPTER 5

Maca For Fertility

One of the most not unusual questions we get is from men and women who've heard about the use of Maca for fertility. Judging from these questions, there's a good misinformation out there regarding the way to use Maca to increase your chances of getting a baby. That's why i decided to put this comprehensive book together.

How The Use Of Maca For Fertility Was Discovered

Maca (Lepidium meyenii) is a root vegetable that grows high in the Andes Mountains. It is in fact the world's highest growing food crop and has grown there naturally for thousands of years. The story of maca and fertility begins when Incan farmers observed how feeding maca roots to their farm animals made them more potent and healthier. With consistent maca feeding, the farmers also noticed that their animals had more and healthier babies.

It wasn't long after that people commenced the usage of maca to increase their own chances of conceiving. Natives of the Andes have long used maca for fertility purposes – and with good success. So much success that it was maca's fertility enhancing properties that first attracted North American and European researchers and doctors to start using it within the 1980s and 1990s.

How Maca Helps Both Male and Female Fertility

Maca is considered one of a few herbs that are believed to be "adaptogens." these special kinds of herbs adapt to a variety of conditions within a given body and help restore it to a healthy balance. Maca in particular works on the endocrine system to balance hormones in both males and females.

Clinical research, some of which are referenced below, have found that using of Black Maca boosts sperm count in men or even increases sperm activity. Similar studies show that female given Maca respond with increased regularity in cycles and less complicated ovulation. Some other result of taking maca is a marked increase in libido for both women and men.

Similarly to balance hormones taking maca also provides excellent nutritional support. Maca is rich in amino acids, phytonutrients, fatty acids, vitamin and minerals. Both women and men who are properly nourished substantially increase the likelihood of conceiving a healthy child.

How To Use Maca for Fertility

In case you decide to use maca for fertility purposes there are numerous things that you have to do and keep in mind in order to maximize your success.

- Use only high quality, fresh, certified organic maca powder. Unfortunately, there are many inferior products on the market that are made from chemically grown maca or from old maca roots that have lost their potency.

- Use the proper quantity of maca. Using Maca for fertility is considered to be a therapeutic utilization and therefore you need to take a therapeutic, always and often.

- Both partners should use maca. For optimum efficiency you and your companion have to be taking Maca. Maca comes with a number of other benefits, so it should to be easy to convince him/her to do so.

- Women should consider using Red Maca for fertility. It is most nutritionally dense form of maca is and also the best for women fertility

- Men should use Black Maca for their fertility. Black Maca has been proven to increase sperm count and sperm motility

- Try cleansing and detox too. Completing an intensive cleansing program will help you get more out of Maca. That's because a good detox will cleanse your intestines and permit more nutrients to be absorbed by body.

- Do not forget getting this natural fertility resource. Similarly, to taking Maca there are many things you can do to increase your chances of a natural conception. The best resource I've seen is referred to as **Pregnancy Miracle**. It's jam pack with natural fertility strategies (along with taking Maca for fertility!)

Some Success Stories

Here are some couples who've reported having success using Maca for fertility.

"We tried a lot of things to get pregnant before we learned about Peruvian Maca in a book on natural fertility. My husband and i started taking it religiously after that. I got pregnant 6 months later and that I'm sure the Maca helped." *Jennifer and Ray Collins, Washington*

"I believe that Maca helped us to conceive naturally when traditional fertility treatments failed. I now have a happy & healthy baby." *Rachel.W, United Kingdom*

"My spouse (wife) and i were together for 7 years before we conceived. The only thing we did differently prior to that was to complete a round of serious detox and to start taking Maca. I'm convinced that Maca played an important part in getting pregnant." *Matt Leonard*

CHAPTER 6

How To Use Maca for Fertility

In case you decide to use maca for fertility purposes there are numerous things that you have to do and keep in mind in order to maximize your success.

- Use only high quality, fresh, certified organic maca powder. Unfortunately, there are many inferior products on the market that are made from chemically grown maca or from old maca roots that have lost their potency.

- Use the proper quantity of maca. Using Maca for fertility is considered to be a therapeutic utilization and therefore you need to take a therapeutic, always and often.

- Both partners should use maca. For optimum

efficiency you and your companion have to be taking Maca. Maca comes with a number of other benefits, so it should to be easy to convince him/her to do so.

- Women should consider using Red Maca for fertility. It is most nutritionally dense form of maca is and also the best for women fertility

- Men should use Black Maca for their fertility. Black Maca has been proven to increase sperm count and sperm motility

- Try cleansing and detox too. Completing an intensive cleansing program will help you get more out of Maca. That's because a good detox will cleanse your intestines and permit more nutrients to be absorbed by body.

- Do not forget getting this natural fertility resource. Similarly, to taking Maca there are many things you can do to increase your chances of a natural conception. The best resource I've seen is referred to as **Pregnancy Miracle**. It's jam pack with natural fertility strategies (along with taking Maca for fertility!)

Some Success Stories

Here are some couples who've reported having success using Maca for fertility.

"We tried a lot of things to get pregnant before we learned about Peruvian Maca in a book on natural fertility. My husband and i started taking it religiously after that. I got pregnant 6 months later and that I'm sure the Maca helped." *Jennifer and Ray Collins, Washington*

"I believe that Maca helped us to conceive naturally when traditional fertility treatments failed. I now have a happy & healthy baby." *Rachel.W, United Kingdom*

"My spouse (wife) and i were together for 7 years before we conceived. The only thing we did differently prior to that was to complete a round of serious detox and to start taking Maca. I'm convinced that Maca played an important part in getting pregnant." *Matt Leonard*

CHAPTER 7

Where To Find And How To Use Maca Root

At this point in time, you're probably wondering: "where can i buy maca?"

Thanks to its growing popularity, maca is broadly available at health stores, pharmacies and even on-line retailer. It can also be found in pill, liquid, powder or extract form. All forms are thought to be equally beneficial, however it's best to buy maca from a quality harvester that guarantees its 100 percent pure maca root powder. Ideally, you should also look for a variety this is raw and organic.

Additionally, maca is categorized based on the color of its roots and is most commonly yellow, black or red. All colors of maca have similar benefits, despite the fact that precise maca types and colors are thought to be more beneficial for certain medical conditions.

Maca tends to have an earthy, barely nutty taste with a hint of butterscotch that works specifically well when added to oatmeal or cereal. The taste may vary based on the type of maca, with black maca being a bit more sour and cream-colored roots having an even sweeter taste. Maca powder can be easily added to smoothies and drinks or mixed into recipes.

Keep in mind that most people prefer not to microwave or warmness their maca powder at high temperatures because the heating method may decrease some of the nutrients.

In the Andes Mountain, locals may consume as much as a pound of dried or fresh maca root daily. Most people supplement with somewhere between one gram to 20 grams daily in powder form.

Despite the fact that there is no official recommended maca powder dosage, it's best to start out with about one tablespoon (in powder shape) daily and work your way up to two to three tablespoons spread throughout the day. Due to the fact maca is known for increasing energy and stamina, many people like to take it before exercising to get a burst of extra energy.

Side Effects

Dietary supplements and drugs affect the body in a similar manner. They can enhance health but sometimes at a price. Some herbs, kava as an example, may cause organ damage, however the side effects associated to Maca appear less intense. An experiment described in the 2008 volume of "Food and Chemical Toxicology" assessed the protection of Lepidium consumption in patients experiencing symptoms of diabetes. Participants acquired either Maca or Placebo for 60 days. This treatment increased diastolic blood pressure. It also increased aspartate transaminase, a caution sign for tissue damage. Both changes were small, and their medical relevance remains unclear. Yet, the general public is urged to await more safety information before taking maca.

About the Author

Dionisia Onio is an Health Researcher ftom Italy who has developed a series of fabulous and highly effective healthful strategies. She applies his knowledge and astonishing perception to analyze the background and underlying causes of various diseases and health related problems affecting people in the world and then designs individualized and totally effective strategies to attain the desired results in solving human related problem with diseases.

Acknowledgments

The Glory of this book success goes to God Almighty and my beautiful Family, Fans, Readers & well-wishers, Customers and Friends for their endless support and encouragements.

www.ingramcontent.com/pod-product-compliance
Lightning Source LLC
Chambersburg PA
CBHW031910200326
41597CB00012B/579